ISBN-13: 978-1537270982
ISBN-10: 1537270982

BISAC: Health & Fitness / Oral Health

Published by

Dr. Emmanuel W. Francis

Dedication

To my beloved wife, Andrea, who successfully raised our children, Ishmael, Denise and Kendra, free from dental disease.

Preface

Dental disease in children is a global healthcare problem which can be eradicated since tooth decay is primarily a preventable disease.

My hope is that parents would benefit from the advice given here to the extent that their children would live healthier, happier lives.

Moreover, families can escape the financial burden brought on by the escalating cost of dental healthcare by following these dental disease prevention tips.

Acknowledgement

I am grateful to the faculty and staff of Meharry Medical College who taught us the importance of Preventive Dentistry in children as an integral component of holistic medicine.

Contents

Prenatal Development

1. Please ensure that your pregnancy is supervised by appropriate medical personnel throughout the course of gestation.
   This includes regular dental treatment after the first trimester to reduce the chance of infection. It is safe, however, to do routine cleanings in the first trimester.

2. Expecting mothers are susceptible to 'pregnancy gingivitis' due to accompanying hormonal changes. Adherence to a strict oral hygiene regimen with routine dental cleanings will help reduce its incidence and severity.

3. Since teeth begin to form at about six (6) weeks in the womb, with mineralization from about the third or fourth month, they are vulnerable to developmental abnormalities months before birth.
Care must be taken to avoid all medications that carry pregnancy warnings about birth defects as these can affect teeth and bone development as well.

4. The enamel which covers the crown of the tooth forms first and is susceptible to medications, especially tetracycline antibiotic which stains developing teeth.

5. Unfortunately, parents must address congenital genetic abnormalities which adversely affect enamel and dentin formation (dysplasia): e.g. Enamelogenesis Imperfecta and Dentinogenesis Imperfecta.

6. Infections in the mother can affect developing teeth with dysplasia or abnormal enamel defects and therefore should be controlled. (Penicillin is usually the antibiotic of choice.)

7. Pregnant women should avoid areas where viral disease outbreaks like measles or Zika occur to protect developing jaws and teeth in the womb.

8. Drinking fluoridated water with a concentration of 1 part per million has been shown to promote the growth of cavity-resistant teeth Too much fluoride, however, is harmful to tooth and bone development.

9. Proper nutrition is essential to teeth development. Balanced meals with a maternal multivitamin and mineral supplement are usually recommended.

Choosing a Dental Home

1. A Dental Home is the dental office or clinic where your child will become one of the family at a very early age.

2. Do not switch dentists at random but allow time for bonding and development of trust.

3. Try to find a dentist reasonably close to where you live.

4. Look for a dentist whose office is child friendly and the team compassionate.

5. Check references and reviews on your dental choice.

6. Take out a health insurance plan
   for your child that includes dental
   benefits from infancy.

7. Keep all appointments and be on
   time, but be patient.

8. Be polite and pleasant, it will reap
   a harvest of love and respect
   wherever you go.

9. Teach your children to be
   hygienic, mannerly and respectful
   to others.

First Dental Visit

1. The American Academy of Pediatric Dentists agrees that the first dental visit should be at age one (1) year.

2. Morning appointments are best for children so plan ahead.

3. Do not change the routine as it relates to sleep and feeding.

4. Keep a smile on your face and avoid emotions of anger, rage, shock and fear as the child can sense these and become anxious.

5. Adopt a pediatric dentist if your personal general dentist is uncomfortable with children.

6. Children with special needs e.g. autism, birth defects, attention deficit, etc. should be referred to a pediatric dentist for management.

7. Avoid self-diagnosis, self-medication, and advice from non-professionals.

8. Be prepared to give a comprehensive medical history on the child including current medication, allergies, operations, hospitalizations, and illnesses.

9. The primary objective of this appointment is to build trust.

Facing Dental Fears

1. Everybody is afraid of something and dentistry presents many possibilities for fear and anxiety.

2. Parents must face their own fears before teaching their children to be fearless.

3. When talking about the dental experience avoid using words that have painful connotations. e.g. instead of needle, stick, shot or injection, use words like pinch or mosquito bite.

4. Keep conversation about dental treatment positive and optimistic with the assurance that all will be well.

5. Do not threaten the child with a visit to the dentist as punishment for bad behavior. This negatively affects efforts to allay fears.

6. Keep a smile on your face, a child can read your fears and become afraid.

7. Don't allow persons who habitually tease children to accompany you on the dental appointment. They can introduce or magnify fears.

8. Avoid screaming at the child and rough draconian tactics for behavior modification. This only creates clamor and confusion.

9. Try to remain concerned but calm.

Brushing & Plaque Removal

1. Plaque is biofilm, an invisible thin layer that forms on all oral tissue surfaces. It is made by and contains bacteria which cause tooth decay and gum disease. Dietary sugars accelerate plaque formation and activity.

2. Brushing is the most effective means of plaque removal.

3. The tongue, palate and gums must be brushed along with the teeth.

4. The first primary teeth begin to erupt at about 6 months and should first be cleaned using a new washcloth until the child can sit up.

5. Start brushing using a soft dry brush with about a pea size amount of toothpaste to mitigate toothpaste ingestion.

6. When plaque is not removed, it accumulates as a calcified deposit which can only be scaled off by professional cleaning.

7. Plaque disclosing products are an excellent aid in exposing invisible plaque for effective removal. These are marketed as chewable tablets or solutions.

8. Between brushings, toothbrushes should be stored in transparent containers as light inhibits bacterial growth.

9. Use light forces when brushing. Only the tips of the bristles are effective in cleaning teeth.

Common Dental Myths

1. A dentist is not really a doctor.
   (This is untrue since their medical
   training makes them 'physicians'
   of the oral cavity.)

2. Baby teeth are unimportant since
   they will be changed anyway.
   (Healthy teeth in childhood are
   essential for growth, general
   health, nutrition, wellness, and the
   development of permanent teeth.)

3. Filling stops toothache.
   (Toothache from decay usually
   indicates the need for pulp therapy
   or extraction to eliminate pain.)

4. Pregnancy causes tooth loss in mothers because of calcium depletion by the fetus.
(Pregnancy does not change the minimum calcium requirement. Tooth loss in pregnancy usually occurs from dental neglect).

5. Oral disease is unrelated to systemic disease.
(There is definite association between heart disease and bacteria in the blood from periodontal (gum) disease.)

6. Aspirin will stop toothache pain when placed in the cavity.
(Aspirin and other over the counter pain relievers act on the brain to affect pain perception, and are useless as topical anesthetics.)

7. A filled tooth cannot decay again.
   (Fillings do not make teeth
   immune to decay. Dietary habits
   and oral hygiene which caused the
   cavity in the first place can make
   it happen again.)

8. Bleaching weakens teeth.
   (This is untrue but sensitivity after
   whitening has occurred)

9. Pregnant mothers should avoid
   dental treatment altogether.
   (Routine dental treatment is safe
   after the first trimester.
   Appointments should short and
   medications administered at the
   lowest therapeutic levels.)

Practical Home Remedies

1. Apply a cold pack and ice chips intraorally within the first 24 hours to reduce inflammatory swelling from trauma.

2. Use a heat pack and warm salt water rinses to reduce swelling from infection. Take prescribed antibiotics only as directed.

3. Use a damp tea bag as pack for troublesome oozing of blood following a dental extraction. (Always notify your dentist if bleeding is a problem)

4. Place oil of cloves, vanilla extract, or garlic in a cavity to reduce pain until you get to the dentist.

5. Sweets stuck in a cavity could cause pain: Brush them out and neutralize the sugar with warm salt water.

6. Avoid eating hard, sweet, or cold things when there is an active cavity: These can trigger a pain reaction.

7. Use an electric toothbrush for children with disability or to encourage compliance.

8. When using hydrogen peroxide as an oral rinse for infection, dilute to 1/3 with water and use intermittently: i.e. four (4) days on, four (4) days off.

9. Do not rinse with hydrogen peroxide or mouthwash following a dental extraction. These adversely affect blood clot formation and hinder post-operative healing.

Dental First Aid

1. It is important to wear protective gloves when working in the mouth to prevent infection and the spread of infectious disease.

2. Preserve a tooth that is knocked out (avulsed) by storing in salt water or milk until a dentist can replant and stabilize it ASAP. Try not to touch or clean the root surface as you could damage root attachment fibers.

3. A tooth that is shifted out of place from impact trauma can be gently repositioned until it can be expeditiously stabilized at the dentist.

4. Apply pressure to any problematic bleeding areas.

5. Topical oral analgesics are helpful in reducing pain from oral lesions that hinder feeding.

6. Take over the counter analgesics for pain. (N.B. Some analgesics like aspirin may exacerbate bleeding so read labels if bleeding accompanies the pain)

7. Seek professional help early. Do not rely on self-diagnosis and advice from non-professionals.

8. Antiseptics like iodine can be applied on wounds to reduce local infection using a saturated cotton tip applicator or medicine dropper.

9. If you suspect a broken jaw, immobilize the jaws together using a head wrap bandage from top to bottom. Seek emergency dental treatment.

Choosing Healthy Snacks

1. The best snacks are raw fresh fruits, vegetables, and nuts. They are low sugar, 'detergent foods' that scrub away plaque from teeth and gums on eating.

2. Always read labels for the sugar, dye, and preservative content of packaged (processed) goods.

3. Avoid being drawn to sugary drinks and snacks by pretty labels and marketing brands.

4. Choose a cold cereal with no added sugar, flavoring, or coloring.

5. Pack a fruit with lunch and have them eat it last to favor plaque reduction while at school.

6. Drink more water. This can help rinse acid promoting sugars off the teeth and prevent decay.

7. No snacks for kids at night after brushing. Bacteria continue to work while you sleep, so don't help them.

8. Have children eat meals on time to avoid between meals snack dependency (munchies).

9. Keep a diet diary for your child noting the frequency of sugar exposures. Get professional help if this diary indicates an addiction to sweets.

Oral Habits & Habits Breaking Appliances

1. Finger, tongue, and other oral habits can cause serious malocclusions (bad bites) without early professional intervention. (Tongue thrusting and thumb sucking are the most common).

2. Tongue thrust is a habit where the child's swallowing pattern does not progress from infantile (absence of erupted teeth) to mature (after teeth erupt). The tongue pushes the anterior teeth forward during swallowing often creating an open bite and loss of incisive (cutting) function.

3. Children suck their thumbs for comfort and calming especially when tired, scared, sleepy or starting pre-school. Most kids stop on their own by age three.

4. Passive sucking is harmless but more rigorous sucking would require professional intervention by age four (4). Parents can help by creating activities to offset habits.

5. Patients presenting with oral habits are probably best managed by a pediatric dentist, or orthodontist, or both if the cases are severe.

6. The objectives of treatment involve removal of the cause, retraining exercises and implementation of mechanical restraining appliances.

7. Fixed habit breaking appliances are preferred over removable ones to ensure patient compliance.

8. Successful treatment may be completed in a few weeks, but other more difficult ones may take months; so be patient.

9. Not all thumb sucking habits are damaging to the teeth and jaw alignment. The parameters to consider are frequency, intensity, and duration.

Conclusion

Dental disease can be prevented and controlled when proactive measures are applied daily from conception as an integral component of universal Healthcare.

The International Dental Federation (FDI) reminds us of the importance of oral health to holistic medicine in their World Oral Health Day (WOHD) - 2016 theme: "It all Starts Here: Healthy Mouth Healthy Body".

The FDI also recommends that we start early, develop good oral habits and "Live Mouth Smart".

It is my hope that this exercise will be a helpful literary resource in simplifying dental health education for parents.

www.ingramcontent.com/pod-product-compliance
Lightning Source LLC
Chambersburg PA
CBHW070246290526
45789CB00004B/1790